AUBREE ECK

Optimal Health Simplified

An Easy Guide to Improve Your Health, Prevent Illness, and Live Vitally

"In health there is freedom. Health is
the first of all liberties."

HENRI FREDERIC AMIEL

Contents

Preface

I am writing this book in hopes of inspiring others to connect the dots and realize the incredible potential we hold to transform our health and lives through conscious choices in our diet and lifestyle. By adopting these simple health practices, you can begin to take your health into your hands and give yourself the opportunity to live a long, healthy, and vibrant life.

Acknowledgement

I would like to thank my dear friend Charlie Anderson for all the hours and care he put into editing my book. I would also like to express my gratitude to my parents, Vince and Kim Eck, for supporting me in pursuing an education in my passion. And I would like to extend an additional heartfelt thank you to my mother Kim, for all of her support and part in editing this book.

I would like to thank all of the scientists, teachers, and the community of functional medicine for discovering and sharing the wealth of knowledge that could change health care for the better. Without your research, teachings, and support we would not have been able to understand the intricacies of the human body and explore innovative approaches to healing. Your tireless dedication to advancing the field of functional medicine has not only educated and empowered countless individuals but also revolutionized the way we approach healthcare.

1

Introduction

Maybe you're reading this book because you want to optimize your health and prevent health issues in the future. Maybe you would like more energy, better focus, to lose that pesky 10 pounds, or to better be able to do the activities you love. It is possible you are here because you recently started having health issues or received a diagnosis. Or maybe you have been dealing with a chronic health issue that no one can solve. Our bodies, just like the Earth, are complex and contain a blueprint for optimal function. It is only when we get in the way of our bodies' natural systems that issues arise. These disruptions can be anything from toxins and improper nutrition to stress and lack of sleep and exercise. If we are to remove these triggers and replace them with what nourishes our body, our body will want to naturally steer back to its default (optimal function). This doesn't usually happen overnight. Just as it takes time to disrupt a system, it takes time for that system to remember its blueprint and heal. Our bodies want to heal, so let's jump in and learn how we can provide our body with the tools it needs to utilize its natural healing capabilities.

2

What is Functional Nutrition and Medicine?

Although the steps towards building and maintaining good health may seem straightforward, unraveling the underlying causes of your symptoms or illness can be a complex journey. That is why finding a practitioner who can help you connect the dots becomes crucial. It ensures you are on the proper healing path. Functional Nutrition and Functional Medicine excel at guiding individuals by addressing the root causes and providing a comprehensive approach to promote overall well-being.

Functional nutrition operates under the foundational belief that Andrea Nakayama, expresses as "Everything is connected. We are all unique. All things matter." Functional Nutritionists and Medicine Practitioners are dedicated to providing every client with a personalized approach, recognizing that each individual's journey towards optimal health is unique. We are focused on finding the root cause of your health symptoms and tailoring the right diet and lifestyle tools to help restore optimal health and function throughout your whole body.

Functional Nutrition is a way out of the cookie cutter approach of our health care system. Often, when you go in to see a doctor, they will listen to your symptoms, order some basic labs, and then calculate a diagnosis based on these bits of information. Treatment usually entails medicine to act as a temporary fix and only addresses the symptoms rather than the cause. This method fails a majority of people, especially those with chronic conditions.The doctors are not necessarily to blame, rather, it is the way our system has been built. Most doctors were provided with shockingly little nutrition education in their medical training. Fortunately, more doctors are starting to seek and incorporate functional medicine, nutrition, and lifestyle training into their practices.

Our bodies operate in a beautifully choreographed dance, maintained and influenced by each intricate system and the communications between them. When outside influences alter or compromise these systems or communications, imbalances occur. If the trigger is not removed and the imbalance persists, we may start to see symptoms and/or disease that can vary in severity and length. Functional Nutrition and Medicine bring together a practice of deep physiological science, intuition, and the open mind to discover the undiscovered.

3

Blood Sugar

Often, when blood sugar is mentioned, our thoughts instinctively turn towards diabetes. While this is a very real and possible outcome of unhealthy blood sugar, it is important to understand that blood sugar impacts EVERY part of our health, and can contribute to diseases and ailments beyond diabetes. Blood sugar affects our hormones, sleep, inflammation, cardiac health, our ability to lose weight, our mental function, and truly every other area of health. Given its significance and role in various health concerns, blood sugar is often one of the first areas of health I assess for every client that comes into my office.

The Wrong Villain in Heart Disease

Fat has long taken the blame for sugar's role in heart disease. This vilification began with the physiologist, Ancel Keys, who sought out to find the answer as to why heart disease was on the rise in America following World War II. Keys traveled the world gathering data and trying to find the correlation between the

American diet and heart disease. He came to the conclusion that dietary fats and cholesterol were to blame, as Americans had a heavy meat and dairy diet. Keys strongly urged the American Heart Foundation to advise Americans to eat less fat. Keys' work became the foundation that led to the U.S Department of Agriculture (USDA) issuing guidelines advising Americans to avoid consuming fats and cholesterol of all kinds.

Unfortunately, Keys' research was highly flawed, leaving out countries like Germany who also had higher fat diets, and lacking proper scientific evidence. Scientists have continued to find holes in his research, yet the myth persists and still impacts the way American doctors and consumers think about fat and heart disease. This misinformation has led many doctors to recommend to their patients to eat less fat. The unfortunate part in suggesting eating less fat is that people often replace it with carbohydrates (sugar), the more common culprit in heart disease.

In the 1950's, scientists were starting to assess the correlation between sugar and heart disease, but because the sugar industry was funding key research, these studies were never publicized. Thankfully, these studies have now come to light and have exposed sugar's role in heart disease.

How is Sugar the Culprit?

There are many ways in which high sugar/carbohydrate consumption and high blood sugar contribute to heart disease risk:

1. **Increase in Advanced Glycation End Products (AGES):** AGES are harmful molecules that form when excess sugar

in the bloodstream attaches to a protein or other molecule. Accumulation of AGES in the bloodstream can contribute to the development and progression of heart disease through inflammation, oxidative stress, endothelial dysfunction, cholesterol modification, and more. AGES increases the production of reactive oxygen species that can damage the cells lining the blood vessels, promoting the development of atherosclerosis.

2. **Increased Blood Pressure**: High sugar and carbohydrate consumption can lead to impaired endothelial function that can result in decreased nitric oxide production. Nitric oxide helps the blood vessels to relax and aids in regulating blood pressure.

3. **Increased Inflammation:** Excess sugar consumption and elevated blood sugar can trigger inflammation in the body. Inflammation increases the risk for atherosclerosis, the formation of plaque, endothelial dysfunction, blood clots, and more.

4. **Increased Oxidation of LDL:** Modification of low-density lipoprotein (LDL) cholesterol. Research has shown that AGES can modify LDL, making it more prone to oxidation. Oxidized LDL is highly inflammatory and can promote the formation of atherosclerotic plaques.

5. **Increased Triglycerides:** Excess carbohydrates are converted into and stored as fat (triglycerides). Excess sugar intake also blocks our bodies from breaking down and utilizing triglycerides. Elevated triglyceride levels are a significant marker for heart disease risk.

Excess carbohydrate intake can also lead to fatty liver disease, promote insulin resistance, lead to obesity, and alter lipid profiles, all of which are risk factors for cardiovascular disease.

The Blood Sugar Roller Coaster:

Many Americans are consuming far too many carbohydrates, mostly in the form of simple or refined carbohydrates (white rice, white breads, sweets, corn syrup/sugars). When we eat a meal imbalanced with too many carbohydrates, our blood sugar spikes. This can result in mood swings, anxiety, brain fog, and increased fat storage. Our body has a narrow window it likes our blood sugar to stay in. When our blood sugar spikes our body overcorrects by secreting excess insulin to bring the sugar into our cells. Now our blood sugar is low, which can cause cravings (for more sugar), fatigue, and brain fog. When our blood sugar is low, our body releases the stress hormone cortisol to try and bring our blood sugar back up. This can turn into a vicious cycle causing crashes, excess stress, and various other health issues down the road.

How Do We Take Control of Our Blood Sugar?

We can avoid the blood sugar roller coaster by balancing our meals with healthy fats, quality proteins, and complex carbohydrates. I will speak more into healthy fats and quality proteins in the Nutrition section of this book. For now, as a simplified guidance, a balanced meal would look like around half of your plate being full of vegetables, about a palm size piece of protein, and the incorporation of healthy fats (these are often already present in a quality animal protein). You can also garnish with healthy fats or add in things like avocado or nuts. If you are going to add in grains or other carbohydrates, I recommend these being a smaller portion of your meal, ideally taking up no more than ⅛ or ¼ of your plate. This is a general guide; if you would like to find out what is best for your body, I recommend working with a nutritionist to find out your ideal macronutrient needs.

***Pro Tip:** if you are going to eat grains I recommend soaking, fermenting, and sprouting your grains before cooking them. One simple way you can do this is by soaking your grains in warm water and adding a tablespoon or so of apple cider vinegar (ACV) or lemon juice. Try to soak them overnight or for at least 7-8 hours, though a short soak is better than none.

Not All Carbohydrates are Created Equal:

All carbohydrates are broken down into sugar or glucose molecules, but the rate at which they enter our bloodstream and the way they impact our physiology differ. Simple carbohydrates are those that are made up of one to two sugar molecules. They are readily digested and quickly absorbed into the bloodstream, often leading to a spike in blood sugar. They can provide a rapid boost of energy. Simple carbohydrates are commonly found in packaged foods and include products like white bread and pasta, fruit juices, table sugar, sodas, and more.

Complex carbohydrates consist of long chains of sugar molecules, which take longer to break down and digest. They provide a steady and sustained release of energy. Complex carbohydrates primarily comprise whole foods found in the produce section and include products such as whole grains, legumes, vegetables, and fruits. They are often high in fiber, vitamins, and minerals, slowing the rate at which the sugars enter our bloodstream, preventing blood sugar spikes, and providing us with more nutrients. By eating more complex carbohydrates and limiting simple and refined carbohydrates, we can keep our blood sugar within a healthy range and supply our body with the vital nutrients for optimal function.

You can also support healthy blood sugar levels by managing stress, getting adequate sleep, and exercising. I will speak more into how these three areas of health affect blood sugar in the upcoming chapters.

4

Nutrition

The nutrients we find in our food are compounds that are required by every body system and function. We use fats to build our cells and fuel our brains, proteins to build muscle and enzymes, sugars to fuel us, magnesium for muscle and nerve function, zinc for supporting our immune system and gut health, and on and on. Each nutrient has many functions. Whenever we become deficient in a nutrient, the functions and pathways that rely on that nutrient become compromised.

How Can You Get Adequate Nutrition?

Organic, Local, and Regenerative Farming

- The sad truth is that our food is becoming less and less nutrient dense. The farming practices we have adopted, such as mono cropping and deep tilling, are depleting our soils and therefore depleting our food. The good news is more farmers are adopting farming practices that heal our lands and increase the health of our food. I had the great opportunity to work for the organic Kern Family Farm in North Fork, California. While working there, I was able to witness how mimicking nature in farming practices was able to create healthier land and therefore more nourishing food. I learned no-till, cover cropping, and other regenerative farming practices. These practices make profound changes such as reducing erosion, creating sustainable lands, increasing organic matter and producing healthier soils. An example from the Kern Family Farm was the increase in earthworm population after adopting regenerative farming practices. Earthworm presence and abundance is indicative of healthy soil. A great way to ensure the highest nutrient density from your food is to buy local, organic, or at best regenerative farming produce and meat, when you can. Growing your own garden is another incredible way to provide yourself with nutrient dense food. Look for good compost, organic and diverse seeds, and organic or high quality soil!

***Pro Tip**: You can find the "dirty dozen" online, a list of what produce is most important to purchase organic. High fat foods, such as nuts and oils, are often good to prioritize, because they store more toxins.

Diversity

- In order to ensure we obtain all essential nutrients, it is important to eat a varied and diverse diet. Seeking out different vegetables, fruits, meats, nuts, seeds, grains, legumes, greens, etc. A great way to diversify is to apply for a CSA (Community Supported Agriculture). You will receive a variety of different produce and food products that will encourage you to branch out, all while advocating for local communities and sustainable eating habits.

Healthy fats

- Cooking with fats: It is important to use fats with high smoke points and cook at low temperatures. Olive oil, though commonly used, is not a good fat to cook with. Olive oil has a low smoke point and is often cooked at a temperature too high. However, olive oil and other fats with low smoke points can provide great health benefits when used without heat such as drizzling over your salad, vegetables, stir frys, etc. When we cook a fat past its smoke point, it oxidizes and releases harmful free radicals. To avoid this, use fats with high smoke points, cook at lower temperatures, sous vide, or use a water sautee and then add the fat after for flavor.

Fats with higher smoke points: Avocado oil, ghee, coconut oil, and butter.

Quality Proteins

- Quality proteins are complete, well sourced, and well prepared. A complete protein contains all of the essential amino acids. Essential amino acids are those that cannot be made by the body and must be obtained through diet. Well sourced proteins are those that are organic, naturally raised, grass-fed, wild caught, and do not contain hormones and antibiotics. Just a reminder that some terms such as natural and free range may not indicate good quality. Natural Grocers and many others have great resources to learn more about labels online.

Complex Carbohydrates and Balanced Meals

- As discussed in the Blood Sugar Chapter, complex carbohydrates contain fiber that can help to slow the rate at which sugar enters the bloodstream, supporting balanced blood sugar levels. This fiber also helps to nourish and support a healthy gut microbiome as well as supporting healthy digestion overall. Complex carbohydrates are also more nutrient dense, supporting healing nutrient levels for optimal health and function.

Food Sensitivities

- We compromise our guts, immune systems, and therefore our whole body when we eat foods we are sensitive to. Healing is nearly impossible if we continue consuming these foods. The main food sensitivities and allergies we see are: gluten, dairy, eggs, soy, seafood, peanuts, and corn. The best way to find out what foods you are sensitive to is through the Elimination Diet. To do this remove all trigger foods, in addition to any foods you think you may be sensitive to, for at least 2 weeks (ideally a month), but most importantly until your symptoms have improved. When you are ready, add in one food at a time and monitor for symptoms. If you develop symptoms when reintroducing a food, remove it from your diet for now. For some, once your gut is healed, you may be able to bring the food back in. I recommend meeting with a nutritionist for support and guidance with this diet. The main two food sensitivities I see in my practice are gluten and dairy.

Gluten and Dairy

- Gluten and dairy, often found in high carbohydrate foods, both have the potential to wreak havoc on our digestion systems, cause inflammation, and can contribute to or exacerbate autoimmunity. More and more people are becoming sensitive to these foods as we see an increase in compromised digestion and gut health. Not everyone needs to remove gluten and dairy, but it can be advantageous to bring awareness to how you feel when you eat them. Do you feel better if you remove or limit them? If your digestion is compromised, I recommend removing these foods until healed. Even in the absence of a food sensitivity gluten and dairy can exacerbate inflammation and digestive issues. As with any food, the type of crop as well as the way they are grown, harvested, and prepared, matter. The type of wheat we grow in America has a higher protein (gluten) content than that in Europe. We also mass produce bread products, often skipping or rushing the fermentation process that aids our body in digesting the bread. This is why people often do better with real sourdough bread that has been made from a starter or breads from European countries. Gluten contains a protein called gliadin that is molecularly similar to other tissue in our body, such as our thyroid tissue. If our immune system has created antibodies for gliadin, and we consume gluten, our immune system may get confused and attack our tissue, as seen in individuals with Hashimoto's and other autoimmune diseases. For those that are highly sensitive or celiac it is imperative that you completely avoid gluten, as even small amounts can cause great harm. As for dairy, many of us stop or significantly decrease the production of the enzyme lactase as we get older, making it hard to break down the sugar called lactose in milk. Additionally, the way our milk is pasteurized and processed kills a lot of the enzymes that would help our digestive systems to break it down. This stress can cause inflammation in the digestive system and throughout the body.

Gluten and Dairy Pro Tips:

1. Gluten can be sneaky, often hiding in sauces, mixed in with burgers, coated on your fries, and may even be found in your cocktail or other beverages. To avoid gluten it is important to read labels and ask your server if your meal contains gluten.
2. Some dairy products are easier to digest than others. Harder cheeses and fermented or cultured dairy products, such as kefir and yogurt, often have lower lactose content and higher levels of beneficial bacteria, making them easier to digest for some individuals.

5

Gut Health

The increasing emphasis on gut health is well-deserved and vital, as it serves as the foundation for overall well-being. Without a healthy gut, the process of healing and enhancing other areas of health becomes significantly challenging, if not impossible.This is where our nutrients are absorbed to then be transported all over the body to be used as fuel and resources for every critical body function. This is also where some neurotransmitters are made, the largest amount of beneficial bacteria reside (microbiome), where we absorb water, rid of many toxins and waste, and much more.

The Microbiome and Probiotics

Did you know that you may have more bacterial cells in your body than your own human cells? Current research believes over half of the cells in our body are bacterial cells. Half human, half bacteria. With this information, it should be no surprise that these bacteria play a major role in our health. We continue to discover new bacteria and the new vital roles that they play in our well-being. The term microbiome refers to all of the microbes that reside on and in our bodies, mostly referenced when discussing the gut microbiome (all of the microbes that live in our gut). We hold an intimate and symbiotic relationship with these microbes. If we take care of them, they will take care of us.

How Does the Gut Microbiome Affect Health?

These microbes that live within our gut produce many beneficial compounds such as:

1. Lactic acid to support optimal pH and healthy microbial balance.
2. Enzymes to aid in breaking down our food and support healthy digestion.
3. Short chain fatty acids such as butyrate, which functions as fuel for supporting healthy colon cells, aids in regulating the immune system, and supports a healthy appetite.
4. Vitamins such as some B vitamins and Vitamin K.
5. Neurotransmitters that influence both the enteric and central nervous systems. A lot of research has come out about the microbiome's role in mental health, especially in anxiety and depression. Research shows that around 90% of our serotonin is made in the gut. Some other neurotransmitters made by gut bacteria are:

- GABA
- Dopamine
- Norepinephrine
- Histamine
- Acetylcholine

Other Benefits of the Microbiome:

- Supports healthy immunity.
- Supports a healthy and balanced inflammatory response.
- Prevents the build-up of harmful bacteria.
- Detoxification.
- Believed to influence healthy blood sugar, skin pH, lung health, hormone levels, and much more.

The Gut and Immunity Connection

Our gut is our first line of internal immune defense. When the gut is functioning properly it acts as a physical barrier to harmful substances.. Research has found that the gut harbors 70-80% of the immune system. IgA is one of the most important immune-supportive proteins in the gut, binding toxins to have them excreted in the stool, as well as calming and modulating inflammation. When our guts become compromised and inflamed our immune systems can begin to overreact and contribute to autoimmune and other immune-related diseases.

Simple Steps to Improve Gut Health and Digestion

1. **Chew food well and slowly** - Digestion starts in our mouth. Chewing aids in the mechanical breakdown of our food, taking the load off of the rest of our digestive system. Our saliva contains enzymes that help with chemical breakdown.
2. **Support stomach acid** - Low stomach acid is becoming very common. Proper stomach acid is vital for proper

digestion and balanced microbial health. Low stomach acid can result in excessive belching and gas, fatigue, heartburn, and headaches. You can boost stomach acid by adding a tablespoon of apple cider vinegar or squeezing some lemon into warm or room temperature water as well as taking some digestive bitters 15-20 minutes before a meal.

3. **Avoid food sensitivities and limit processed foods** - These foods wreak havoc on your digestive system and can cause inflammation throughout your body.

4. **Eat more fiber** - Prebiotic foods are fibers that cannot be broken down by our digestive system and are instead fermented by beneficial bacteria, resulting in the production of beneficial compounds, such as short chain fatty acids. Fiber also helps to speed the digestive transit time and aids in the removal of harmful bacterias from the colon. It is important to get both soluble fiber (sweet potatoes, broccoli, beans, carrot, etc.) and insoluble fiber (celery, beans, cauliflower, etc). For optimal health, get your fiber from a variety of vegetables, grains, and greens.

5. **Exercise** - Exercise aids in healthy digestion by strengthening abdominal and core muscle tone as well as increasing blood flow to digestive muscles to support peristalsis, or the movement of our food through the digestive tract.

6. **Take probiotics** - As we talked about above, a healthy microbiome is essential for good health. Due to our lifestyle, farming practices, and over-sanitization, most of us are not getting enough exposure to healthy bacteria. Taking probiotic supplements along with eating prebiotic fibers can help us to foster a healthy microbiome.

7. **Drink Water** - For healthy digestive tissue, proper break-

down, absorption, and transportation of vital nutrients.

6

Sleep

We all know the difference of how we feel after a good versus a poor night's sleep. Our mood, energy, and focus all change dramatically. Sleep has been a mystery and an area of interest to scientists for a long time. We have started to learn more about how sleep impacts our health and will only continue to discover its vital role in our health.

How Sleep Affects Our Health

Compromised sleep can:

1. Increase cortisol, the stress hormone, putting our sympathetic nervous system in overdrive. This can impact our stress levels, hormones, blood sugar, and digestion.
2. Impacts blood sugar levels to the point of causing a pre-diabetic state. Increased cortisol causes a release of glucose into the blood, and on top of that, a lack of sleep inhibits our bodies' ability to take up the sugar in our blood stream.
3. Compromise our immune system. Sleep deprivation can alter the production of important immune-regulating

cells and molecules, such as cytokines, and increase pro-inflammatory signaling. Compromised sleep has been linked to a dysregulated immune system, decreased ability to fight infection, immune threats, and heal, as well as increased inflammation.

4. Increase the hunger protein ghrelin, causing us to feel hungrier than we really are and potentially over eat.

5. Cause weight gain and decrease our ability to lose weight.This is in part due to the increase in ghrelin resulting in overeating. Sleep deprivation can also lead to compromised metabolism, increased stress, and decreased growth hormone levels, all of which are associated with obesity.

6. Contribute to or exacerbate anxiety and depression. Studies have shown that sleep deprivation increases systemic inflammation and can negatively alter the gut microbiome, both of which are linked to mental health. Additionally, our cognition and ability to deal with stressors is significantly decreased, which can exacerbate mental health issues.

7. Increase the chance for cardiac disease. I have seen this over and over again in my practice. Many of my cardiac clients have reported spending a large portion of their life getting less than 5 or 6 hours of sleep most nights. Too much time spent in the sympathetic state from poor sleep can result in increased heart rate and strain our blood vessels. As stated above, compromised sleep also affects blood sugar and stress, two major contributors to heart disease. Look back at the Blood Sugar chapter to learn more about sugar's role in heart disease.

8. Strong correlations between lack of sleep and increased

risk of cancer, Alzheimers, type 2 Diabetes, heart disease, and more.

How Much Sleep Should We Get?

Research indicates that receiving any less than 7 hours of sleep can start to have a significant and far-reaching impact on our health. Most of us in the medical community agree that 7-8 hours of sleep a night is optimal for health. Studies are also pointing to potential health risks for those sleeping more than 9 hours. If you are sleeping more than 9 hours it is important to know why. There may be other areas of your health compromised that are causing you to need or desire this much sleep. Some causes for needing more than 9 hours are: depression, poor sleep or sleep apnea, restless legs, hormone or blood sugar issues, chronic fatigue, and more. I hear all too many clients tell me they do not need more than 5 hours or they are just a person that needs 10 and they always have been. While I do believe in biological individuality, our bodies do all work in similar ranges. You may feel okay with 5 hours because this has been your normal baseline for some time, so you do not actually know how good you could feel if you were getting 7-8 hours consistently. You may feel okay, but research shows your body is being harmed/compromised by this sleep deprivation, and you may be increasing your chance of disease later on. If you feel your body just needs 10 hours, there may be an underlying health concern that has not yet been discovered.

Sleep Hygiene

As you can see, there are many factors that may be contributing to poor sleep. If you are experiencing trouble sleeping, feeling tired upon waking, or feel that you need more than 8 or 9 hours, I recommend meeting with a nutritionist or functional medicine practitioner that can help you to discover the root of your health and sleep issues.

Tools to help you get a better night's sleep

1. Aim for 7-8 hours nightly
2. Adopt a consistent sleep schedule, to the best of your ability.
3. Stay away from screens the hour or 2 before you go to bed. Look into wearing blue light glasses if you are going to be looking at a screen after dark.
4. Make sure your room is completely dark and cool enough.
5. Wind down and relax as bed time approaches. Do some yoga, read a book, take a bath/shower, meditate, or bring in your favorite way to relax.
6. Avoid eating close to bedtime, especially sugar or high carbohydrate meals. If you need to eat close to bedtime eat a protein-rich snack.
7. Go outside and get some sunlight in your eyes right when you wake. This has worked very well for many of my clients with sleep issues. Note: Do not look directly at the sun, of course!
8. Try to save your bed for sleep and sexual activities/intimacy only.

***Pro Tip:** If you have a hard time falling asleep, make a calming sleep playlist or use sleep meditations. Insight Timer, Waking Up, and Calm are all great apps for meditations.

7

Water

Our bodies are made up of around 60% water. With more than half of our body weight being water it should be no surprise that it plays a huge role in our health and well-being. Following oxygen, it is the first thing our body dies without. Yet even with this knowledge, most people are not consuming optimal amounts of water and many health care professionals overlook this simple solution to their patients' health concerns. Dehydration can significantly impact all areas of our health.

How Water/Hydration Affects Our Health

1. **Detoxification** -Aids in transporting toxins and waste out of the body, while supporting healthy bowel transit time. Healthy bowel transit times decrease the amount of time our colon cells are exposed to our waste and the harmful components within. Increased exposure can lead to colon damage and increase our risk for diseases such as

colon cancer.

2. **Immunity** -Water plays an important role in helping to transport our immune cells to injured and infected areas. It also aids in the removal of harmful toxins as well as bacterial and viral threats.

3. **Digestion** -Supports metabolism, lubrication of the gastrointestinal tract membranes, and proper transportation of nutrients to all cells.

4. **Body Temperature Regulation**-Water is essential for regulating our body temperature as we are exposed to extreme heat and cold, fever, and exercise.

5. **Some other areas affected by proper hydration:**

- Skin health and appearance
- Joint and spinal health
- Brain health
- Weight loss
- Energy
- Tissue and organ health
- Every area of health directly or indirectly

How Much Water Should We Drink?

- The general rule of thumb is to drink about half of your body weight in ounces daily and maintain clear urine. Your water needs will vary and increase based on physical exertion, consuming dehydrating substances (like alcohol), illness, infections, etc.
- Drink plain water. Seltzer waters, teas, etc. should not count as a part of your water intake.
- Some ways to help remind yourself to drink enough water:

- Buy one of the big jugs that has water consumption goals based on the time of the day and stay on track.
- Set reminder alarms on your phone.
- Have a water bottle with you at all times.
- Tally how many water bottles/cups you have had.

***Pro Tip:** If you find flavor is what is deterring you from drinking water, I recommend adding lemon, cucumber or fruit to your water to give it a healthy flavor boost!

8

Exercise/Physical Activity

E xercise and physical activity has always been a hot topic in health and for good reason. It is one of the most important actions we can take for our health alongside sleeping and nutrition.

Health Benefits of Exercise and Physical Activity

1. **Immune support:** Exercise aids in the circulation of our lymph, helping our bodies to clear the toxins and harmful compounds within. Exercise also supports blood circulation, supporting the transport of important immune cells and nutrients throughout the body.
2. **Digestive health**: Exercise aids in peristalsis and increased transit time throughout the bowels.
3. **Blood sugar**: Exercise increases insulin sensitivity, supporting healthy blood sugar levels and decreasing our risk for type 2 diabetes and other health issues.
4. **Mental health**: Exercises release chemicals such as endor-

phins that can help to improve your mood and feel more relaxed. Exercise can help improve symptoms of anxiety and depression while also helping you better cope with stress.

5. **Better focus and brain health:** Exercise stimulates the release of important compounds such as brain-derived neurotrophic factor that help to improve and maintain proper structure and function of the brain. Exercise can help us to focus, learn, and better apply current knowledge.

6. **Sleep:** Exercise can help you better fall asleep, stay asleep, and spend more time in deep restorative sleep. Time of day may be important. Exercising at night can stimulate the brain and cause a rise in core body temperature that may interfere with falling asleep. Exercising in the morning or afternoon may be more advantageous for those who have trouble falling asleep.

7. **Support sexual health/ performance:** For men, exercise can help with arousal and aid in decreasing the risk of erectile dysfunction due to its support in circulation. For women, the increased circulation can help increase clitoral stimulation and vaginal lubrication.

8. **Bone, muscle, and structural health**: Exercise, along with proper nutrition, helps to create stronger and denser bones and muscles. This increased strength helps to protect joints from injury. Exercise is also shown to decrease joint pain and stiffness.

9. Exercise and physical activity also helps to prevent many diseases such as heart disease and type 2 diabetes as well as significantly increase our life span.

Move Often

Research is starting to find that prolonged inactivity can inhibit us from receiving the health and metabolic benefits of our exercise. If you were to go for a 5 mile run in the morning and then sit all day, you may not be receiving the full potential benefits from your earlier 5 mile run. Research is showing it is very important to limit our sedentary hours and make sure we squeeze in movement and physical activity in between our sedentary hours to receive the full potential of exercise benefits and decrease our risk for disease and injury.

Exercise Practices For Optimal Health

Physical activity will and should look different for everyone. We all have different physical needs and abilities based on our age and current health. It is important to tune into your body and find a balance of challenging yourself without pushing yourself too far. If you are currently experiencing adrenal fatigue or compromised hormonal health, excessive strenuous activity may worsen your symptoms. If you are experiencing serious health or cardiac issues, consult your primary practitioner about what level of exercise is appropriate for you.

Start slow and build up

If you are seeking to start exercising and currently do not have a practice, start slow and build up intensity and frequency over time. You may start with 20 minute walks and simple at-home exercises. If you have a current exercise practice and are looking to ramp it up, slowly continue to increase the intensity and frequency, making sure you are challenging yourself but not depleting yourself.

Rest

Proper rest is just as important as the exercise itself. Exercise is stressful on our bodies, and if that stress is not met with proper rest, we may tax our adrenals, which can lead to chronic fatigue and hormonal imbalances. Rest also allows our muscles to strengthen and decreases our risk for injury. Listen to your body and take the proper rest you need. It can be helpful to break up your week with different forms and target areas of exercises to balance exercise and rest for each body part.

Movement

Bring in movement throughout your day. Physical activity does not always have to look like a crazy workout. Break up your sedentary work day by using a standing desk, going for a walk on your breaks, or finding some other form of movement that speaks to you.

Balance

It is important to balance your exercise routine with cardio, strength training, mobility and flexibility exercises.

Cardio or aerobic exercise: Cardio, as implied in the name, is important for your cardiac health, supporting a healthy heart rate, blood pressure and circulation. It is also important for sleep, immunity, brain health, blood sugar and mental health. Some forms of cardio are:
    *Running
    *Swimming
    *Biking
    *Skiing/ touring
    *Speed walking/Brisk walking

*Hiking

Strength/ resistance training: Strength or resistance training is a form of exercise that increases muscular strength and endurance by exercising a specific muscle or muscle group against an external resistance. This training can be performed using bodyweight exercises, like push-ups or squats, or with exercises that use equipment like resistance bands, dumbbells, kettlebells, barbells, etc., according to the National Academy of Sports Medicine (NASM). Benefits of strength training include:

*Increased muscle tone and strength.

*Increased bone density and health with a decreased risk for developing osteoporosis.

*Supports cardiac, metabolic, brain, and emotional health.

Flexibility/ Mobility: Flexibility and mobility exercises are important for keeping your muscles and joints happy to decrease your risk of injury. These exercises allow your joints to move in their full range of motion, decrease stiffness and pain, increase circulation, and support strength and physical performance. You can increase flexibility and mobility through practices like yoga, pilates, static and dynamic stretching (static stretching is best done after exercise), myofascial release using things like tennis balls, and at-home mobility exercises.

Nutrition and Exercise

Every function in our body is made possible by the nutrients we consume and produce. Whenever we put added stress on our bodies, such as exercise, our nutrient needs are increased.

It is important to restore our bodies with nutrient-dense foods following exercise.

Carbohydrates

Carbohydrates are our body's preferred fuel source. It is important to replenish our bodies' glycogen stores (the storage form of glucose) after exercise. It is often thought that this is best done with simple carbohydrates that are rapidly absorbed into the bloodstream. However, research has shown that it is best to refuel with complex carbohydrates. Complex carbohydrates are more nutrient dense, helping us to replenish nutrient stores beyond carbohydrates and have been found to result in a greater amount of muscle glycogen synthesis. Refer back to the Blood Sugar chapter to learn the difference between simple and complex sugars. To best restore glycogen synthesis it is ideal to refuel with your post-workout snack within 30 minutes of exercise.

Protein

Protein is essential for rebuilding your muscles and replenishing your body. Refer to the Nutrition chapter to learn about quality proteins. It is important to include protein in your post-workout snack to replenish and support healthy blood sugar levels. You can aim for your post-workout snack to have 1 gram of protein for every 4 grams of carbohydrate.

Fat

Fat is an important metabolic fuel for endurance exercise and also plays many crucial roles in essential functions and optimal health. During prolonged exercise, especially at low-intensity, our body will convert to using fat as a fuel source. It is important to consume healthy fats, which you can learn more about in the Nutrition chapter. Fat intake should comprise at least 15-30% of your daily nutrition. I recommend working with a nutritionist to determine your individual fat needs.

9

Stress

Stress may be one of the most important and overlooked areas of health. While we may not have control over all the stressors that come into our lives, we do have the ability to adopt and utilize tools and practices that can better help us cope with the stressors. It is important to note that not all stress is bad. Acute stress, such as exercise or a sudden event, can be beneficial for our bodies. It is only when stress becomes chronic or is not resolved in an appropriate amount of time that it can wreak havoc on our bodies.

How does stress affect our health?

Stress increases the release of the hormone cortisol. Cortisol can affect nearly every organ system in the body through glucocorticoid receptors. Cortisol influences our blood sugar, blood pressure, inflammation, metabolism, sleep, hormonal health, and more. I will touch on just a few.

<u>Blood sugar:</u> When a surge of cortisol is released, it signals

35

our bodies to release more sugar into the blood for emergent use. This is helpful if we need to run from a lion, but not so helpful in the event that someone cuts us off in traffic. Stress can also make our cells more resistant to insulin, the hormone responsible for shuttling glucose into cells and regulating blood sugar. Chronic stress can lead to unhealthy blood sugar levels, increasing our risk for various diseases.

<u>Inflammation:</u> Acute stressors can actually temporarily decrease inflammation. It is chronic or frequent release of cortisol that can cause an overactive immune system and lead to an imbalanced inflammatory response. Additionally cortisol's ability to lead to chronically elevated blood sugar levels can also contribute to increased inflammation throughout the body. Chronic inflammation is at the root of many, if not most, of the chronic diseases and health issues that plague us today.

<u>Hormonal Health:</u> Cortisol is a glucocorticoid hormone released by the adrenal glands. Hormones are essentially messengers that coordinate different functions throughout the body. A hormone imbalance is where there is too little or too much of one or many hormones in the bloodstream. As with any system in our body, hormones are intricately connected and influence one another. Elevated cortisol can unfavorably impact other hormones such as estrogen, testosterone, thyroid hormone and more. Hormonal imbalances can cause an array of health issues that can seriously impact quality of life.

How can we take control over our stress?

You can start by removing the stressors you have control over in your life. We often have more control over this than we would like to believe. Can you better prioritize your schedule and be more efficient? Are the relationships in your life becoming sources of stress? If so, consider engaging in constructive conversations, creating personal boundaries, or even removing toxic relationships to promote your well-being. Check in with yourself often about what is causing your stress and what is in your power to change.

Bring in practices for healthy coping.

1. Seek out support: coaching, talk therapy, psychedelic assisted psychotherapies, eye movement desensitization and reprocessing therapy, etc.
2. Practice mindfulness and living in the present moment: yoga, meditation, mindfulness apps, journaling, podcasts.
3. Bring in other activities that help you to relax: exercise, art, music, walking, baths, etc.
4. Work on changing your mind's reaction to events or situations by redirecting or reframing. When you notice yourself becoming frustrated or stressed, can you pause, evaluate if you are making the situation a bigger deal than it is? Is your worry or reaction necessary, can you take an action or think of the situation in a way that will cause less stress?
5. BREATHE! Our breath is one amazing tool we can use to bring ourselves out of the flight or fight mode and back into rest and digest. When you feel yourself becoming stressed, use deep breaths to help bring you back down. One simple breath technique you can adopt is the box breath. The box breath is a breathing technique that involves inhaling, holding the breath, exhaling, and holding

the breath again, each for an equal count of time. Using a count of 4 can be a great place to start.

10

Conclusion

Although these practices I have shared are important for optimal health, I have come to find that balance is always the answer. While it is important to adopt healthy practices and take care of your body, it is also still important to make sure you are enjoying life and not taking it too seriously. I have seen too many become too serious over their health and burn themselves. This approach can lead to increased unhappiness and stress. I have also been here myself and learned the importance of prioritizing happiness too. I do believe the balance of good health and enjoying life exists, it is just a learning curve. Be patient with yourself as you adopt these new diet and lifestyle practices. It is not an all or nothing, and adopting any of these practices is a step towards better health. Make the changes you can at a rate that is approachable for you. See how you can make them enjoyable and where you can bring in the balance.

I hope you are closing this book having gained a profound understanding of your body and how to care for it, enabling you to experience the vibrant and fulfilling life you truly deserve. I wish you a new sense of empowerment, now knowing the control you have over your health through your own diet and lifestyle choices.

Live well and take care of each other!

11

About the Author

Aubree started battling health issues in her first years of life. The doctors referred to her as a medical mystery, as they could never arrive at a diagnosis or find solutions. Through Aubree's long, defeating, and complicated health journey she began to discover natural healing alternatives that brought her hope and true healing. These discoveries opened her eyes to our bodies' natural healing capabilities. Aubree was immediately captivated by the concept that simple diet and lifestyle tools could be the answer to debilitating and overlooked health issues. She became passionate about becoming an expert in the field, and that passion drove her to learn as much as she could about the human body and natural alternatives. She was determined to help others unravel their complex health puzzles and reclaim their lives.

Aubree is the founder of Healing Roots Nutrition where she is the lead Functional Nutrition and Lifestyle Practitioner. She is an herb and supplement expert, mental health coach, educator, and a published author with a long history of her own health challenges. Through applying her own nutrition and lifestyle education, Aubree is now living her life pain free and in remission from her other health challenges. Her life mission is now to give others the same hope and opportunity

12

Sources

Harmon, W. (2022, December 31). *How To Soak & Cook Whole Grains (+grain cooking chart)*. Traditional Cooking School by GNOWFGLINS. https://traditi onalcookingschool.com/food-preparation/grain-cooking-ch art/

GIORDANA VOGEL. (2022, November 15). *The differences between American & European wheat/gluten.* De La Heart. https://www.delaheart.com/blogs/food/the-differences-bet ween-american-european-wheat-gluten#:~:text=Fact%3A%2 0American%20wheat%20is%20higher,thus%20lower%20in% 20gluten%20content.

MS, C. K. (2022). The gluten-thyroid connection. *Chris Kresser.* https://chriskresser.com/the-gluten-thyroid-connection/co mment-page-11/

Anderson, L., MD. (2019). Who needs more sleep? We do! *Thriven Functional Medicine Clinic.* https://thrivenfunctionalm

edicine.com/who-needs-more-sleep-we-do/

Colten, H. R. (2006). *Extent and health consequences of chronic sleep loss and sleep disorders*. Sleep Disorders and Sleep Deprivation - NCBI Bookshelf. https://www.ncbi.nlm.nih.gov/books/NBK19961/

Eck, A. (n.d.). *Nutrition | Healing Roots Nutrition | Fort Collins*. Healing Roots. https://www.healingroots-nutrition.com/

Eck, A. (2021, January 3). *How dehydration impacts your health*. Healing Roots. https://www.healingroots-nutrition.com/post/how-dehydration-impacts-your-health

Fu, J., Zheng, Y., Gao, Y., & Xu, W. (2022). Dietary fiber intake and gut microbiota in human health. *Microorganisms, 10*(12), 2507. https://doi.org/10.3390/microorganisms10122507

Akins, J. D., Crawford, C. H., Burton, H. M., Wolfe, A. S., Vardarli, E., & Coyle, E. F. (2019). Inactivity induces resistance to the metabolic benefits following acute exercise. *Journal of Applied Physiology, 126*(4), 1088–1094. https://doi.org/10.1152/japplphysiol.00968.2018

Exercise | New England Center for Functional Medicine | Functional Medicine in New England. (2020, September 3). https://necfunctionalmedicine.com/2020/09/03/exercise/

Mahaffey, K. (n.d.-b). *Resistance training Exercises & Concepts you should use*. https://blog.nasm.org/resistance-training

Fry, A., & Dr. Rehman, A. (2022). Obesity and sleep. *Sleep Foundation.* https://www.sleepfoundation.org/physical-healt h/obesity-and-sleep

Barnard, D. (2019). Why is mobility training important for your health? *Inspire Fitness for Wellbeing.* https://www.inspire-fitness.com.au/blog/2018/07/why-is-mobility-training-imp ortant-for-your-health/

Professional, C. C. M. (n.d.). *Cortisol.* Cleveland Clinic. https://my.clevelandclinic.org/health/articles/22187-cortiso l

Alyssa. (2020). The connection between stress & your hor-mones. *Capital Women's Care of Rockville.* https://rockvilleob gyn.com/blog/the-connection-between-stress-your-hormon es/#:~:text=When%20high%20cortisol%20levels%20lower,H eavy%20or%20frequent%20periods

Yang, D.-F., Huang, W.-C., Wu, C. W., Huang, C.-Y., Yang, Y.-C. S. H., & Tung, Y.-T. (2023, March). *Acute sleep deprivation exacerbates systemic inflammation and psychiatry disorders through gut microbiota dysbiosis and disruption of circadian rhythms.* ScienceDirect. Retrieved July 15, 2023, from https://www. sciencedirect.com/science/article/pii/S0944501322003329

Garbarino, S., Lanteri, P., Bragazzi, N. L., Magnavita, N., & Scoditti, E. (2021). Role of sleep deprivation in immune-related disease risk and outcomes. *Communications Biology,* *4*(1). https://doi.org/10.1038/s42003-021-02825-4

Ending the war on fat. (2014, June 12). *Time*. https://time.com/2863227/ending-the-war-on-fat/

MS, C. K. (2022b). Here's the research on sugar and health. *Chris Kresser*. https://chriskresser.com/heres-the-research-on-sugar-and-health/

Hegab, Z., Gibbons, S., Neyses, L., & Mamas, M. A. (2012). Role of advanced glycation end products in cardiovascular disease. *World Journal of Cardiology*, 4(4), 90. https://doi.org/10.4330/wjc.v4.i4.90

www.ingramcontent.com/pod-product-compliance
Lightning Source LLC
Chambersburg PA
CBHW031334250726
48656CB00005B/2117